CRANIAL OSTEOPATHY

A Complete Guide On Unveiling The Power Within And Bridging Science And Holistic Healing

WALTER ZYAIRE

No part of this book may be reproduced, stored in a retrieval system, or transmitted in any form or by any means, electronic, mechanical, photocopying, recording, or otherwise, without the express written permission of the author, with the exception of small extracts in critical reviews or articles.

DISCLAIMER

based on the author's research and understanding at the time of publishing, it could not reflect the most recent developments or practices in the treatment area. The publisher and the author both disclaim all liability for the accuracy, completeness, or use of the material in this book. Readers bear full responsibility for the decisions and actions they choose in light of the information presented in this book.

TABLE OF CONTENTS

ABOUT THE BOOK

The thorough guide "Cranial Osteopathy: Exploring the Foundations and Applications" explores the nuances of cranial osteopathic procedures. The book starts by giving readers a thorough introduction to cranial osteopathy, including its goals, boundaries, and intended audience. This introduction lays the groundwork for a detailed examination of the topic.

The significance of comprehending cerebral anatomy is emphasized. Readers obtain a deep understanding of the anatomical underpinnings essential for successful cranial osteopathic therapy through in-depth talks on skull structure, cranial sutures, cerebrospinal fluid dynamics, and the relationships between the brain and nervous system.

The book provides an in-depth historical development of cranial osteopathy, highlighting its inception, trailblazers, and the progression of its tenets. This background information enhances the reader's comprehension of the subject and provides a framework for discussing important ideas in cranial osteopathic philosophy.

The book explains the fundamentals of cranial osteopathic treatment, with a focus on the importance of palpation, soft touch, and knowledge of inherent motion and the main respiratory mechanism. The section on somatic dysfunction in the cranial field helps the reader understand basic concepts that are necessary for therapeutic application on a deeper level.

The phase covers clinical assessment, which is investigated using a variety of thorough methods such as palpation techniques, patient history and interviews, and observation. This basis equips professionals to diagnose patients in the context of cranial osteopathy with efficacy.

Cranial osteopathic procedures are discussed and divided into two categories: indirect and direct methods. Subsections provide practitioners with a practical application guide by describing articulatory procedures, soft tissue approaches, and specialized techniques like frontal lift and cranial base release.

Cranial osteopathy is applied in a wider range of fields, such as sports medicine, pediatrics, and the treatment of certain ailments. This thorough investigation highlights the applicability and usefulness of cranial osteopathy in a range of medical settings.

The book discusses integration with traditional medicine, highlighting teamwork with other medical specialties and encouraging evidence-based methods in the sector.

The book, the author frankly discusses difficulties and disagreements, addressing disputes and complaints while offering a forum to clear up misunderstandings about cranial osteopathy. This well-rounded viewpoint advances a thorough comprehension of the subject.

"Cranial Osteopathy: Exploring the Foundations and Applications" is essentially a crucial tool that provides both new and seasoned practitioners with a comprehensive and deep understanding of cranial osteopathy, from its historical origins to its modern applications, guaranteeing a well-rounded and knowledgeable approach to practice.

CHAPTER ONE

OVERVIEW OF CRANIAL OSTEOPATHY

THE SYNOPSIS OF CRANIAL OSTEOPATHY

A comprehensive approach to medicine, cranial osteopathy emphasizes the connections between the structure and function of the spine, the skull, and the body as a whole. Osteopathy, which was developed in the late 19th century by Dr. Andrew Taylor Still, emphasizes the body's capacity for self-healing and maintaining balance.

A subspecialty of osteopathic medicine called cranial osteopathy explores the complex dynamics of the skull and how they relate to a person's general health.

The foundation of cranial osteopathy is the idea that the skull is a dynamic system with intrinsic movement rather than a fixed structure. Experts in this field think that involuntary motion—tiny motions within the skull bones—is essential to preserving health and wellness.

The goal of cranial osteopathy is to identify and correct any limitations or imbalances in these movements, which can be connected to a variety of medical conditions. The method is mild and uses accurate palpation and manipulation techniques to support the body's natural healing processes.

GAINING KNOWLEDGE OF CRANIAL ANATOMY

A thorough understanding of cranial anatomy is essential to comprehending cranial osteopathy. The intricate bone structure known as the skull supports the face structures while enclosing and shielding the brain.

The frontal, parietal, temporal, and occipital bones are among the many bones that make up the cranium. These bones articulate through joints called sutures. The dynamic character of the cranial system is reflected in these sutures, which permit small movements.

HEAD STRUCTURE

The complex structure of the skull accomplishes more than just protecting the brain. The cranial vault safeguards the important cerebral structures, whereas the facial bones support the sense organs. Cranial osteopathy acknowledges that to guarantee the unhindered operation of the nervous system and general physiological equilibrium, it is critical to preserve the ideal alignment and mobility of these bones.

HEAD SUTURES

The numerous skull bones are joined by fibrous junctions called cranial sutures. Cranial sutures are not like other bodily joints in that they are made to allow for very little movement, but movement nonetheless. Cranial osteopathy practitioners believe that constrictions or strains in these sutures can affect CSF flow and impair the natural movements of the skull. At the core of cranial osteopathic practice is the application of mild manipulative methods to address these constraints.

THE DYNAMICS OF CEREBROSPINAL FLUID

The clear, colorless fluid that surrounds and nourishes the brain and spinal cord is called cerebrospinal fluid, or CSF. The dynamics of CSF are crucial in cranial osteopathy. The healthy circulation and absorption of CSF are critical to the preservation of the nervous system's structure and functionality. To enhance the body's self-regulatory mechanisms, cranial osteopaths use their talents to evaluate and, if necessary, modify the flow and distribution of CSF.

BRAIN-NERVE SYSTEM RELATIONSHIPS

One of the main ideas of cranial osteopathy is the complex relationship that exists between the cranial structures and the central nervous system. Professionals understand that abnormalities in cranial mobility can affect neurological processes and may be linked to a variety of health problems. Cranial osteopathy seeks to improve the way the brain and nervous system operate by treating limitations in the cranial bones and sutures. This promotes general health and well-being.

Cranial osteopathy provides a distinct viewpoint on medical care by highlighting the interaction of cranial architecture, physiological dynamics, and the body's natural capacity for healing. Through gentle, hands-on approaches, practitioners aim to optimize health and promote balance by understanding the minute changes within the skull and their implications for the nervous system.

CHAPTER TWO

THE EVOLUTION OF CRANIAL OSTEOPATHY THROUGHOUT HISTORY

HISTORY AND PIONEERS

The field of osteopathic medicine includes cranial osteopathy, which dates back to the late 1800s. This therapeutic technique has its roots in the work of Dr. Andrew Taylor Still, the founder of osteopathic medicine. The pioneering concepts of Still promoted a holistic approach to healthcare by highlighting the interdependence of the body's structure and function. Dr. William Garner Sutherland, his pupil, advanced the ideas that would later become the cornerstone of cranial osteopathy.

The discoveries that Dr. Sutherland made during his investigation into the complexities of the cranial bones were revolutionary. He postulated that the skull's bones showed delicate, rhythmic movements rather than being inflexible during the beginning of the 20th century. This idea went against accepted anatomical wisdom and gave rise to the cerebral rhythmic impulse (CRI) concept. Sutherland's contributions, which emphasized the importance of the skull and its connection to the body's general health, set the foundation for the specialized discipline of cranial osteopathy.

PRINCIPLES OF CRANIAL OSTEOPATHY: AN EVOLUTION

Cranial osteopathy has changed throughout the years as its practitioners improved and extended its fundamental ideas. In the beginning, the mobility of the skull bones and the CRI were the main points of interest.

Practitioners became aware of the wider ramifications of these rhythmic movements as the field advanced. The concepts extended to include the entire body, taking into account the interdependence of all body systems and tissues, not only the skull.

One of the main ideas of cranial osteopathy is the primary respiratory mechanism or PRM. According to this holistic viewpoint, the central nervous system's natural motion, or CRI, affects and reflects an individual's general health. Practitioners gained the ability to feel these delicate motions and decipher them as signs of the body's innate capacity for self-healing and self-regulation.

IMPORTANT IDEAS IN THE PHILOSOPHY OF CRANIAL OSTEOPATHY

The core ideas of cranial osteopathic philosophy set it apart from other therapeutic philosophies. An essential concept is the notion of innate self-healing. Practitioners hold the belief that the body has an inherent capacity to preserve equilibrium and well-being, and their job is to support and strengthen this self-healing mechanism.

The idea that structure and function are interdependent is another important one. According to cranial osteopathy, the body is seen as one system in which problems in one area can have a significant impact on the body as a whole. It is the goal of practitioners to maximize the body's overall function by treating constraints and imbalances in the cranial and spinal tissues.

Moreover, cranial osteopathy emphasizes the significance of customized treatment plans. Practitioners customize their care for each patient, taking into account their particular anatomy, past medical history, and current state of health. The larger osteopathic principles of treating the patient as a whole rather than just treating symptoms are consistent with this patient-centered attitude.

The innovative concepts of Dr. Andrew Taylor Still and the ensuing contributions of Dr. William Garner Sutherland are largely responsible for the historical development of cranial osteopathy.

CHAPTER THREE

FUNDAMENTALS OF CRANIAL OSTEOPATHIC MEDICINE

LIGHT CONTACT AND FEELING

The emphasis on delicate touch and probing is fundamental to the cranial osteopathic treatment philosophy. Professionals use a very delicate, highly attuned tactile sense to evaluate the minute rhythms and motions of the cranial system. Because cranial osteopathy recognizes that the cranial structures respond to gentle manipulations, its approach to touch is gentle and non-intrusive. This method makes it easier to identify minute variations in the fluid dynamics, tissue texture, and general cranial rhythm.

Practitioners seek to identify any limitations or imbalances in the cranial structures through gentle touch and palpation. By identifying regions of tension, compression, or dysfunction, the hands-on evaluation assists the osteopath in creating a customized treatment plan. To facilitate a responsive and cooperative healing process, the therapeutic touch in cranial osteopathy is an essential component of building a relationship between the practitioner and the patient's cranial system.

THE PRIMARY RESPIRATORY MECHANISM AND INHERENT MOTION

The core tenets of cranial osteopathic theory are intrinsic motion and the basic respiratory mechanism. It suggests that the entire body, including the skull, moves in a rhythmic manner that is different from the cycles of breathing and heartbeat. This innate movement is thought to be an expression of the body's innate vitality and ability to self-regulate.

The principal mechanism of respiration is based on the oscillation of CSF fluid and the mutual movement of the cranial bones. It is believed that the dynamic interaction of the brain, spinal cord, and sacrum is responsible for this faint, regular pulsing. Cranial osteopaths think that several health problems might arise from abnormalities or limitations in this main breathing mechanism. To maximize the body's self-healing mechanisms, therapy focuses on restoring the harmonious flow of cerebrospinal fluid and encouraging the balanced mobility of cranial bones.

SOMATIC IMPAIRMENT WITHIN THE CRANIAL DOMAIN

Anomalies or imbalances in the musculoskeletal and connective tissue systems of the skull are referred to as somatic dysfunction in the cranial field. Cranial osteopathy recognizes that these dysfunctions can result from stress, trauma, or other circumstances that impact the body's general health and functionality. To detect somatic dysfunction, which might show up as changed tissue texture, asymmetry, or restricted motion, practitioners use their probing abilities?

Gentle, manual approaches are used to treat somatic dysfunction in the cranial field to regain appropriate alignment and mobility.

Cranial osteopaths work to improve these dysfunctions to support the body's natural ability to heal and self-regulate. The comprehensive methodology of cranial osteopathic medicine acknowledges the interdependence of diverse physiological systems and underscores the significance of reestablishing equilibrium to maximize general health and welfare.

CHAPTER FOUR

CLINICAL EVALUATION IN ORTHOPAEDICS

PATIENT BACKGROUND INFORMATION AND CONSULTATION

In cranial osteopathy, clinical assessment entails a thorough examination of the patient that takes into account several ideas, including observation, palpation techniques, patient history and interview, and diagnostic approaches. These components are essential to comprehending the patient's situation and creating a successful treatment strategy.

Clinical assessment is fundamentally based on the patient's history and interview. Osteopaths inquire about the medical background, way of living, and particular concerns of their patients. This procedure aids in determining plausible reasons for the issues that are presented as well as comprehending the context of general health.

Additionally, osteopathic physicians can build rapport with patients during interviews, fostering a cooperative and knowledgeable therapeutic alliance.

TECHNIQUES FOR PALPATION AND OBSERVATION

Another crucial component of clinical assessment in cranial osteopathy is observation. Practitioners closely monitor the posture, gait, and general body mechanics of their patients. Visual clues can offer important insights into possible dysfunctional or imbalanced areas. Finding minor indicators that could support the evaluation and treatment process is made easier by keeping an eye on the patient in a variety of positions and activities.

Palpation techniques are essential to cranial osteopathy because they allow practitioners to evaluate the quality and mobility of tissues, especially in the cranial and sacral areas, with their hands. Osteopaths can identify regions of tension, limitations, and asymmetries in the body through the expert use of palpation. Experts in light touch can detect irregularities or disturbances in cranial and sacral motion, as well as evaluate the rhythm of the cerebrospinal fluid.

METHODS FOR DIAGNOSING CRANIAL OSTEOPATHY

In cranial osteopathy, diagnostic methods comprise combining data from palpation, observation, and patient history to create a diagnosis. Osteopaths use their understanding of anatomy, physiology, and biomechanics to comprehend how the body functions as a whole and its innate capacity for self-regulation. Cranial osteopathy employs a holistic approach to diagnosis, viewing the body as a dynamic system in which dysfunction in one part can have an impact on the whole.

Additionally, to evaluate the natural motion of the cranial bones and associated tissues, cranial osteopaths may use specialized cranial assessment methods, such as cranial rhythmic impulse (CRI) evaluation. Using a hands-on method enables practitioners to examine the general health and vitality of the craniosacral system as well as identify subtle motions.

 Clinical evaluation in cranial osteopathy is a complex procedure that includes palpation techniques, observation, patient history and interview, and diagnostic methods. Osteopaths can better understand their patients' conditions and customize treatment plans to support their utmost health and well-being by using a holistic approach. The goals of cranial osteopaths are to support the body's natural healing process and restore equilibrium with expert examination procedures.

CHAPTER FIVE

OSTEOPATHIC CRANIAL TECHNIQUES

METHODS WITHOUT DIRECT EXPERIENCE

In the context of cranial osteopathic methods, indirect techniques emphasize a delicate and nuanced manipulation of the cranial structures. These approaches are distinguished by a sophisticated comprehension of the body's innate capacity for self-regulation and recovery. Instead of forcing forceful corrections, practitioners using indirect approaches concentrate on engaging the body's natural motion and facilitating its tendencies. This method is in line with the osteopathic theory, which holds that the body has a natural capacity to preserve equilibrium and health.

SOFT TISSUE METHODS

In cranial osteopathy, soft tissue techniques entail evaluating and manipulating the muscles, fascia, and ligaments that surround the cranium. By addressing tension and constraints within these structures, soft tissue methods seek to enhance circulation and movement. To relieve tension and promote the best possible functioning of the soft tissues, practitioners could apply mild pressure, stretches, or myofascial release techniques. Cranial osteopathy's incorporation of soft tissue techniques acknowledges the interdependence of the body's components and the influence of soft tissue health on general health.

SPEAKING METHODS

In cranial osteopathy, articulatory treatments concentrate on the joints or articulations that connect the cranial bones. These methods use little motions to improve the cranial bones' balance and mobility. Articular techniques are intended to promote natural movements and restore optimal joint function, as opposed to direct treatments, which require delivering force to specific locations. To promote mobility and reduce limitations, practitioners carefully evaluate the range of motion in cranial joints and use mild manipulations. The focus on articulatory procedures is consistent with the larger osteopathic philosophy of maximizing structural alignment to facilitate the body's self-healing mechanisms.

The holistic approach of cranial osteopathy is embodied by indirect procedures, soft tissue approaches, and articulatory techniques. These methods emphasize a patient-centered and gentle approach to addressing imbalances within the cranial region. Through these sophisticated therapeutic approaches, practitioners hope to improve general health and well-being by recognizing the body's ability to self-regulate and appreciating the interdependence of all body structures.

STRAIGHTFORWARD METHODS

Using certain manual forces to treat limitations or dysfunctions in the cranial bones and related tissues is known as "direct techniques" in cranial osteopathy.

By restoring the skull's natural motion and equilibrium, these procedures seek to improve general health and well-being. In cranial osteopathy, Frontal Lift and Cranial Base Release are two well-known direct procedures.

RELEASE OF THE CRANIAL BASE

The cranial base—the region where the skull and spine meet—is the focus of the Cranial Base Release. This area is essential for the nervous systems and many physiological systems' correct operation. To relieve tension and constraints in the tissues surrounding the cranial base, the osteopath uses mild pressure and manipulative techniques during the Cranial Base Release procedure.

By improving the cerebrospinal fluid flow and regaining normal cranial bone movement, this procedure seeks to strengthen the body's self-healing capabilities.

FRONT-END LIFT

Another direct method in cranial osteopathy that targets the frontal bone of the skull is called Frontal Lift. In addition to forming the forehead, the frontal bone helps to shape the eye sockets. Using precise and controlled manual forces, the osteopath addresses any limitations or imbalances in the frontal bone by performing a Frontal Lift. The goal of this procedure is to improve the alignment of the cranial structures and lessen stress on the connective tissues. Frontal Lift may aid in better blood flow, lower stress levels, and increased brain function by promoting the best possible movement in the frontal bone.

Since both Cranial Base Release and Frontal Lift involve manual manipulation to target specific parts of the skull, they are excellent examples of direct treatments. To diagnose and treat dysfunctions, these approaches call for a sensitive touch and a deep understanding of cranial anatomy.

Practitioners employ precise forces that support the body's natural ability to heal and maintain equilibrium by drawing on their understanding of the interconnection of cranial components.

In the holistic approach to osteopathy, direct cranial osteopathic treatments such as Cranial Base Release and Frontal Lift are essential. Through the restoration of cranial mobility and balance, practitioners hope to achieve optimal health and well-being by focusing on the complex components of the skull and their linked roles.

CHAPTER SIX

UTILISATIONS FOR CRANIAL OSTEOPATHY:

PAEDIATRIC APPLICATIONS

In pediatrics, cranial osteopathy has proven to be a useful tool as it provides a gentle and non-invasive means of addressing a range of health issues in young patients. According to cranial osteopathy practitioners, minor movements of the cranial bones have an impact on an individual's general health and well-being. This idea is especially important when treating pediatric patients. For example, birth-related stresses may occur in infants and impact their cranial and musculoskeletal tissues. The goal of cranial osteopathy is to reduce these tensions and encourage ideal growth and functionality.

In pediatric patients, practitioners stress the significance of identifying and treating any limitations or imbalances in the cranial bones, face bones, and related soft tissues. It is thought that this method may help with problems including colic, trouble nursing, and sleep abnormalities in babies. Cranial osteopaths use gentle manual techniques to help the musculoskeletal system regain its balance. This can help the body's natural ability to recover and self-regulate, which can be especially helpful in the delicate setting of pediatric care.

OSTEOPATHY OF THE CRANIUM IN SPORTS MEDICINE

Cranial osteopathy has garnered attention in the field of sports medicine because of its potential benefits in enhancing athletic performance and managing musculoskeletal problems in athletes. Athletes frequently have a range of medical difficulties, such as sprains, imbalances, and injuries that can affect their performance. A comprehensive strategy that takes into account the cranial structures as well as the overall musculoskeletal system is provided by cranial osteopathy.

Sports medicine professionals may incorporate cranial osteopathy into a comprehensive treatment plan to promote tissue mobility, optimize biomechanical function, and hasten the healing process. Practitioners seek to optimize neuro-musculoskeletal function by correcting cranial and musculoskeletal abnormalities. This may lower the chance of injury and improve overall sports performance. Because cranial osteopathy is non-invasive and adheres to the concepts of fostering natural healing and restoring equilibrium within the body, athletes value its non-invasive character.

CRANIAL OSTEOPATHY IN THE MANAGEMENT OF PARTICULAR ILLNESSES

Cranial osteopathy is used to treat a variety of distinct diseases in a range of patient demographics. The treatment of nervous system issues, including temporomandibular joint (TMJ) problems, tension headaches, and migraines, is one prominent topic. It is believed by practitioners that little movements of the cranial bones might affect the neurological system's function and the flow of cerebrospinal fluid, which can help relieve various diseases.

Furthermore, cranial osteopathy is used to treat disorders of the digestive and respiratory systems. The mild methods of cranial osteopathy can help patients with respiratory conditions like nasal congestion or asthma by enhancing respiratory function and discharge. In a similar vein, practitioners can utilize these concepts to address digestive issues by highlighting the relationship between the musculoskeletal system and the digestive organs.

Cranial osteopathy expands its applications into a variety of healthcare domains, showcasing its adaptability in treating pediatric issues, supporting sports medicine, and offering substitute methods for treating certain ailments. Throughout various uses, the fundamental idea of reestablishing equilibrium and supporting the body's self-regulation processes is still prevalent.

CHAPTER SEVEN

COMBINING TRADITIONAL AND MODERN MEDICINE

COLLABORATIVE STRATEGIES WITH OTHER MEDICAL SPECIALTIES

Collaborative techniques involving different healthcare professionals have become increasingly popular in the field of integrative medicine. The understanding that many healthcare methods might work in concert to improve patient outcomes has resulted in a rise in interdisciplinary cooperation.

Integrating alternative therapies and holistic approaches is becoming more acceptable in conventional medicine, which is focused on evidence-based practices and pharmaceutical interventions. The delivery of comprehensive care involves a collaboration between physicians and other healthcare professionals, including physical therapists, dietitians, psychologists, and chiropractors.

The partnership promotes a more comprehensive knowledge of patients' health by accounting for psychological and lifestyle issues in addition to physical symptoms. A more individualized and patient-centered style of treatment is made possible by this team-based approach, in which professionals with different backgrounds pool their knowledge to meet the particular requirements of each patient. Improved patient outcomes are the final result of healthcare professionals exchanging knowledge and expertise to ensure a more thorough assessment and treatment plan.

EVIDENCE-BASED CRANIAL OSTEOPATHIC PRACTICES

In both traditional and alternative medicine, cranial osteopathy—a manual therapy technique that focuses on manipulating the skull and its related structures—has drawn attention. Although cranial osteopathy's introduction into traditional medicine has drawn criticism, its supporters contend that evidence-based procedures validate its effectiveness in specific clinical situations. Studies have looked into how cranial osteopathy affects ailments like musculoskeletal discomfort, dysfunction of the temporomandibular joint (TMJ), and migraine headaches.

Supporters of cranial osteopathy stress how critical it is to recognize and honor the body's innate capacity for self-healing and self-regulation. They contend that mild adjustments to the cranial bones and tissues might affect physiological processes in the body, hence improving balance and reducing a range of symptoms. It is important to remember, though, that not all members of the medical profession agree with the findings in favor of cranial osteopathy.

Evidence-based techniques are incorporated into cranial osteopathy through rigorous study, adherence to scientific methods, and peer evaluation of the interventions. Researchers in conventional medicine and cranial osteopaths working together can help develop a more sophisticated knowledge of the circumstances in which this manual therapy may be helpful. This point where ancient manual therapies meet modern research methods is a prime example of how integrative medicine is developing: evidence-based approaches work as a link between conventional and alternative modalities to provide patients with the best care possible.

CHAPTER EIGHT

DIFFICULTIES AND DEBATES

COMMENTS AND DISCUSSIONS

Within the medical profession, cranial osteopathy—an alternative therapy that manipulates the skull and its underlying structures—has generated discussion and controversy. A main area of dispute is that there is little empirical data to prove the effectiveness of cranial osteopathy. Opponents contend that there is little scientific evidence to support the theoretical underpinnings of this treatment, which highlights the minute motions of the cranial bones and their alleged effects on general health.

The discussion also encompasses the more general issue of whether cranial osteopathy belongs in the mainstream of medicine or should be used as a stand-alone treatment. Critics contend that it is difficult to defend the use of cranial osteopathy in conjunction with evidence-based medical treatments due to the practice's scant empirical backing and lack of a well-established scientific foundation. However, supporters assert that by emphasizing the body's self-regulating systems, their holistic approach to healing gives supplementary advantages that can improve general well-being.

The uniformity and standardization of cranial osteopathy procedures have also drawn criticism. The credibility of the field has been questioned by some due to inconsistent training and practice. Critics contend that the safety and efficacy of cranial osteopathy procedures may be jeopardized in the absence of evidence-based recommendations and standardized practices.

DISPELLING MYTHS REGARDING CRANIAL OSTEOPATHY

Even though cranial osteopathy has been criticized, certain frequent misconceptions about it need to be addressed and clarified. The idea that cranial osteopathy entails violently manipulating the bones of the skull is one common misconception. Cranial osteopaths use soft, non-invasive methods to improve the cranial bones' inherent rhythmic motions, which in turn helps the body feel more balanced.

Regarding the range of problems that cranial osteopathy may treat, there is another fallacy. Although advocates may propose an extensive array of uses, it is imperative to recognize that cranial osteopathy is not a cure-all.

Evidence for its efficacy is frequently restricted to particular ailments, such as musculoskeletal problems or particular kinds of headaches. It is easier to control expectations and foster a more realistic perception of the possible benefits of cranial osteopathy when one is aware of its varied breadth.

The arguments and objections raised by cranial osteopathy highlight the necessity of continued study, harmonization, and candid communication among physicians.

Even though there are still certain difficulties, dispelling myths and promoting a thorough knowledge of this complementary therapy might help forward the conversation about its place in medicine.

CHAPTER NINE

PROSPECTS FOR FUTURE DEVELOPMENTS

THE SYNOPSIS OF CRANIAL OSTEOPATHY

Within the field of Cranial Osteopathy, the field is always changing due to continuing study and developments. There has been an increase in scientific investigation and critique of traditional cranial osteopathy, which is based on the ideas presented by Andrew Taylor Still. To give a better evidence-based knowledge of cranial osteopathy's impact on the craniosacral system, recent studies have descended into the physiological mechanisms underpinning the treatment.

A prominent field of study is the neurophysiological underpinnings of cranial osteopathy. Electroencephalography (EEG) and functional magnetic resonance imaging (fMRI) are two neuroimaging techniques that have been used to study alterations in brain activity and connectivity related to cranial osteopathic manipulative procedures. By clarifying the effects of these interventions on the central nervous system, these investigations hope to provide insight into the potential therapeutic mechanisms of cranial osteopathy.

Our comprehension of the mechanical components of cranial osteopathy has also been greatly improved by developments in biomechanical modeling and simulation. To gain insight into the stresses and strains involved in osteopathic manipulations, computational models simulate the interactions between various anatomical systems. This kind of research helps to improve methods and treatment plans, which in turn helps to increase the accuracy and effectiveness of cranial osteopathic therapies.

Furthermore, research on cranial osteopathy is placing an increasing amount of emphasis on personalized medicine. Investigations into genetic and epigenetic variables are being conducted to comprehend individual differences in therapy response. By customizing cranial osteopathic therapies to each patient's unique needs, this technique has the potential to improve outcomes and move the field closer to patient-centric care.

NEW METHODOLOGIES AND APPROACHES

New methods and approaches are developing as cranial osteopathy progresses, broadening the treatment toolkit that professionals can employ. Integrative techniques are becoming more and more popular. These approaches combine cranial osteopathy with other complementary treatments like yoga, acupuncture, or mindfulness. This holistic viewpoint gives patients a thorough and multifaceted approach to health by acknowledging the connection between physical and mental well-being.

Pediatric cranial osteopathy has seen a rise in attention in recent years. Recent research points to its possible advantages in treating newborn colic, torticollis, and plagiocephaly. The main goals of this field of study are to explore the long-term impact of early treatments on developmental outcomes and to refine methodologies appropriate for the pediatric population.

Furthermore, technological developments have opened the door for creative cranial osteopathy techniques. Applications of augmented reality (AR) and virtual reality (VR) are being investigated as ways to boost practitioner training and increase patient involvement. With the help of these immersive learning experiences and visualizations, osteopathic manipulative procedures and the craniosacral system can be understood more intuitively.

A dynamic interaction between current research and developing practices characterizes the future directions in cranial osteopathy. To meet the various needs of patients, the sector is changing towards a more evidence-based and individualized strategy that makes use of scientific breakthroughs and adopts a holistic viewpoint.